My
Daily Food
Log

This log belongs to

____

Today:	Weeklies:	Balance:	

Breakfast:

Snack:

Lunch:

Snack:

Supper:

Total:

<table>
<tr><td>Today:</td><td>Weeklies:</td><td>Balance:</td></tr>
</table>

Breakfast:

Snack:

Lunch:

Snack:

Supper:

Total:

Today:	Weeklies:	Balance:	

Breakfast:

Snack:

Lunch:

Snack:

Supper:

| | Total: | |

Today:	Weeklies:	Balance:

Breakfast:

Snack:

Lunch:

Snack:

Supper:

Total:

| Today: | Weeklies: | Balance: |

Breakfast:

Snack:

Lunch:

Snack:

Supper:

Total:

| Today: | Weeklies: | Balance: |

Breakfast:

Snack:

Lunch:

Snack:

Supper:

Total:

Today:	Weeklies:	Balance:	

Breakfast:

Snack:

Lunch:

Snack:

Supper:

Total:

| Today: | Weeklies: | Balance: |

Breakfast:

Snack:

Lunch:

Snack:

Supper:

Total:

<table>
<tr><td>Today:</td><td>Weeklies:</td><td>Balance:</td><td></td></tr>
</table>

Breakfast:

Snack:

Lunch:

Snack:

Supper:

Total:

Today:	Weeklies:	Balance:

Breakfast:

Snack:

Lunch:

Snack:

Supper:

Total:

Today:	Weeklies:	Balance:	

Breakfast:

Snack:

Lunch:

Snack:

Supper:

Total:

Today:	Weeklies:	Balance:

Breakfast:

Snack:

Lunch:

Snack:

Supper:

Total:

| Today: | Weeklies: | Balance: | |

Breakfast:

Snack:

Lunch:

Snack:

Supper:

Total:

Today:	Weeklies:	Balance:	

Breakfast:

Snack:

Lunch:

Snack:

Supper:

| | Total: | |

Today:	Weeklies:	Balance:	

Breakfast:

Snack:

Lunch:

Snack:

Supper:

| | Total: | |

Today:	Weeklies:	Balance:	

Breakfast:

Snack:

Lunch:

Snack:

Supper:

Total:

Today:	Weeklies:	Balance:	

Breakfast:

Snack:

Lunch:

Snack:

Supper:

Total:

Today: Weeklies: Balance:

Breakfast:

Snack:

Lunch:

Snack:

Supper:

Total:

Today:	Weeklies:	Balance:	

Breakfast:

Snack:

Lunch:

Snack:

Supper:

| | Total: | |

<table>
<tr><td>Today:</td><td>Weeklies:</td><td>Balance:</td></tr>
</table>

Breakfast:

Snack:

Lunch:

Snack:

Supper:

Total:

Today:	Weeklies:	Balance:	

Breakfast:

Snack:

Lunch:

Snack:

Supper:

Total:

Today:	Weeklies:	Balance:	

Breakfast:

Snack:

Lunch:

Snack:

Supper:

Total:

Today:	Weeklies:	Balance:	

Breakfast:

Snack:

Lunch:

Snack:

Supper:

Total:

Today:	Weeklies:	Balance:

Breakfast:

Snack:

Lunch:

Snack:

Supper:

Total:

Today:	Weeklies:	Balance:	

Breakfast:

Snack:

Lunch:

Snack:

Supper:

Total:

| Today: | Weeklies: | Balance: |

Breakfast:

Snack:

Lunch:

Snack:

Supper:

Total:

| Today: | Weeklies: | Balance: |

Breakfast:

Snack:

Lunch:

Snack:

Supper:

Total:

| Today: | Weeklies: | Balance: |

Breakfast:

Snack:

Lunch:

Snack:

Supper:

Total:

| Today: | Weeklies: | Balance: | |

Breakfast:

Snack:

Lunch:

Snack:

Supper:

Total:

Today:	Weeklies:	Balance:

Breakfast:

Snack:

Lunch:

Snack:

Supper:

Total:

Today:	Weeklies:	Balance:	

Breakfast:

Snack:

Lunch:

Snack:

Supper:

| Total: | |

| Today: | Weeklies: | Balance: |

Breakfast:

Snack:

Lunch:

Snack:

Supper:

Total:

Today:	Weeklies:	Balance:	

Breakfast:

Snack:

Lunch:

Snack:

Supper:

| | Total: | |

Today:	Weeklies:	Balance:	

Breakfast:

Snack:

Lunch:

Snack:

Supper:

Total:

Today:	Weeklies:	Balance:

Breakfast:

Snack:

Lunch:

Snack:

Supper:

Total:

Today:	Weeklies:	Balance:

Breakfast:

Snack:

Lunch:

Snack:

Supper:

Total:

Today:	Weeklies:	Balance:	

Breakfast:

Snack:

Lunch:

Snack:

Supper:

Total:

<table>
<tr><td>Today:</td><td>Weeklies:</td><td>Balance:</td><td></td></tr>
</table>

Breakfast:

Snack:

Lunch:

Snack:

Supper:

Total:

Today:	Weeklies:	Balance:	

Breakfast:

Snack:

Lunch:

Snack:

Supper:

Total:

<table>
<tr><td>Today:</td><td>Weeklies:</td><td>Balance:</td><td></td></tr>
</table>

Breakfast:

Snack:

Lunch:

Snack:

Supper:

Total:

<table>
<tr><td>Today:</td><td>Weeklies:</td><td>Balance:</td><td></td></tr>
</table>

Breakfast:

Snack:

Lunch:

Snack:

Supper:

Total:

| Today: | Weeklies: | Balance: |

Breakfast:

Snack:

Lunch:

Snack:

Supper:

Total:

Today:	Weeklies:	Balance:	

Breakfast:

Snack:

Lunch:

Snack:

Supper:

Total:

Today:	Weeklies:	Balance:

Breakfast:

Snack:

Lunch:

Snack:

Supper:

Total:

Today:	Weeklies:	Balance:	

Breakfast:

Snack:

Lunch:

Snack:

Supper:

Total:

Today:	Weeklies:	Balance:	

Breakfast:

Snack:

Lunch:

Snack:

Supper:

Total:

| Today: | Weeklies: | Balance: | |

Breakfast:

Snack:

Lunch:

Snack:

Supper:

Total:

| Today: | Weeklies: | Balance: |

Breakfast:

Snack:

Lunch:

Snack:

Supper:

Total:

Today:	Weeklies:	Balance:	

Breakfast:

Snack:

Lunch:

Snack:

Supper:

Total:

Today:	Weeklies:	Balance:	

Breakfast:

Snack:

Lunch:

Snack:

Supper:

Total:

| Today: | Weeklies: | Balance: | |

Breakfast:

Snack:

Lunch:

Snack:

Supper:

Total:

<table>
<tr><td>Today:</td><td>Weeklies:</td><td>Balance:</td><td></td></tr>
</table>

Breakfast:

Snack:

Lunch:

Snack:

Supper:

Total:

| Today: | Weeklies: | Balance: |

Breakfast:

Snack:

Lunch:

Snack:

Supper:

Total:

Today:	Weeklies:	Balance:	

Breakfast:

Snack:

Lunch:

Snack:

Supper:

Total:

Today:	Weeklies:	Balance:	

Breakfast:

Snack:

Lunch:

Snack:

Supper:

| Total: | |

Today:	Weeklies:	Balance:	

Breakfast:

Snack:

Lunch:

Snack:

Supper:

Total:

| Today: | Weeklies: | Balance: | |

Breakfast:

Snack:

Lunch:

Snack:

Supper:

Total:

| Today: | Weeklies: | Balance: |

Breakfast:

Snack:

Lunch:

Snack:

Supper:

Total:

Today:	Weeklies:	Balance:	

Breakfast:

Snack:

Lunch:

Snack:

Supper:

Total:

<table>
<tr><td>Today:</td><td>Weeklies:</td><td>Balance:</td></tr>
</table>

Breakfast:

Snack:

Lunch:

Snack:

Supper:

Total:

Today:	Weeklies:	Balance:	

Breakfast:

Snack:

Lunch:

Snack:

Supper:

Total:

Today:	Weeklies:	Balance:

Breakfast:

Snack:

Lunch:

Snack:

Supper:

Total:

Today:	Weeklies:	Balance:	

Breakfast:

Snack:

Lunch:

Snack:

Supper:

Total:

Today:	Weeklies:	Balance:

Breakfast:

Snack:

Lunch:

Snack:

Supper:

Total:

Today:	Weeklies:	Balance:	

Breakfast:

Snack:

Lunch:

Snack:

Supper:

Total:

| Today: | Weeklies: | Balance: |

Breakfast:

Snack:

Lunch:

Snack:

Supper:

Total:

Today:	Weeklies:	Balance:	

Breakfast:

Snack:

Lunch:

Snack:

Supper:

Total:

Today:	Weeklies:	Balance:

Breakfast:

Snack:

Lunch:

Snack:

Supper:

		Total:

Today:	Weeklies:	Balance:	

Breakfast:

Snack:

Lunch:

Snack:

Supper:

Total:

Today:	Weeklies:	Balance:	

Breakfast:

Snack:

Lunch:

Snack:

Supper:

Total:

| Today: | Weeklies: | Balance: |

Breakfast:

Snack:

Lunch:

Snack:

Supper:

Total:

Today:	Weeklies:	Balance:	

Breakfast:

Snack:

Lunch:

Snack:

Supper:

| | Total: | |

Today:	Weeklies:	Balance:	

Breakfast:

Snack:

Lunch:

Snack:

Supper:

	Total:	

| Today: | Weeklies: | Balance: |

Breakfast:

Snack:

Lunch:

Snack:

Supper:

Total:

<table>
<tr><td>Today:</td><td>Weeklies:</td><td>Balance:</td><td></td></tr>
</table>

Breakfast:

Snack:

Lunch:

Snack:

Supper:

Total:

| Today: | Weeklies: | Balance: |

Breakfast:

Snack:

Lunch:

Snack:

Supper:

Total:

<table>
<tr><td>Today:</td><td>Weeklies:</td><td>Balance:</td></tr>
</table>

Breakfast:

Snack:

Lunch:

Snack:

Supper:

Total:

Today:	Weeklies:	Balance:

Breakfast:

Snack:

Lunch:

Snack:

Supper:

Total:

Today:	Weeklies:	Balance:

Breakfast:

Snack:

Lunch:

Snack:

Supper:

Total:

<table>
<tr><td>Today:</td><td>Weeklies:</td><td>Balance:</td></tr>
</table>

Breakfast:

Snack:

Lunch:

Snack:

Supper:

Total:

Today: | Weeklies: | Balance:

Breakfast:

Snack:

Lunch:

Snack:

Supper:

Total:

Today:	Weeklies:	Balance:

Breakfast:

Snack:

Lunch:

Snack:

Supper:

Total:

Today:	Weeklies:	Balance:	

Breakfast:

Snack:

Lunch:

Snack:

Supper:

Total:

<table>
<tr><td>Today:</td><td>Weeklies:</td><td>Balance:</td></tr>
</table>

Breakfast:

Snack:

Lunch:

Snack:

Supper:

Total:

| Today: | Weeklies: | Balance: | |

Breakfast:

Snack:

Lunch:

Snack:

Supper:

Total:

<table>
<tr><td>Today:</td><td>Weeklies:</td><td>Balance:</td></tr>
</table>

Breakfast:

Snack:

Lunch:

Snack:

Supper:

Total:

Today: Weeklies: Balance:

Breakfast:

Snack:

Lunch:

Snack:

Supper:

Total:

Today:	Weeklies:	Balance:

Breakfast:

Snack:

Lunch:

Snack:

Supper:

Total:

Today:	Weeklies:	Balance:	

Breakfast:

Snack:

Lunch:

Snack:

Supper:

Total:

Today:	Weeklies:	Balance:	

Breakfast:

Snack:

Lunch:

Snack:

Supper:

Total:

Today:	Weeklies:	Balance:	

Breakfast:

Snack:

Lunch:

Snack:

Supper:

Total:

Today:	Weeklies:	Balance:

Breakfast:

Snack:

Lunch:

Snack:

Supper:

Total:

Today:	Weeklies:	Balance:	

Breakfast:

Snack:

Lunch:

Snack:

Supper:

Total:

Today:	Weeklies:	Balance:

Breakfast:

Snack:

Lunch:

Snack:

Supper:

Total:

Today: Weeklies: Balance:

Breakfast:

Snack:

Lunch:

Snack:

Supper:

Total:

Today:	Weeklies:	Balance:

Breakfast:

Snack:

Lunch:

Snack:

Supper:

Total:

<table>
<tr><td>Today:</td><td>Weeklies:</td><td>Balance:</td><td></td></tr>
</table>

Breakfast:

Snack:

Lunch:

Snack:

Supper:

Total:

<table>
<tr><td>Today:</td><td></td><td>Weeklies:</td><td></td><td>Balance:</td><td></td></tr>
</table>

Breakfast:

Snack:

Lunch:

Snack:

Supper:

Total:

Today:	Weeklies:	Balance:	

Breakfast:

Snack:

Lunch:

Snack:

Supper:

Total:

Today:	Weeklies:	Balance:	

Breakfast:

Snack:

Lunch:

Snack:

Supper:

Total:

Today:	Weeklies:	Balance:	

Breakfast:

Snack:

Lunch:

Snack:

Supper:

Total:

Today:	Weeklies:	Balance:

Breakfast:

Snack:

Lunch:

Snack:

Supper:

Total:

Today:		Weeklies:		Balance:	

Breakfast:

Snack:

Lunch:

Snack:

Supper:

Total:

Today:	Weeklies:	Balance:

Breakfast:

Snack:

Lunch:

Snack:

Supper:

Total:

Today:	Weeklies:	Balance:	

Breakfast:

Snack:

Lunch:

Snack:

Supper:

Total:

Today:	Weeklies:	Balance:

Breakfast:

Snack:

Lunch:

Snack:

Supper:

Total:

Today:	Weeklies:	Balance:	

Breakfast:

Snack:

Lunch:

Snack:

Supper:

Total:

| Today: | Weeklies: | Balance: |

Breakfast:

Snack:

Lunch:

Snack:

Supper:

Total:

Today:	Weeklies:	Balance:

Breakfast:

Snack:

Lunch:

Snack:

Supper:

Total:

Today:	Weeklies:	Balance:	

Breakfast:

Snack:

Lunch:

Snack:

Supper:

Total:

| Today: | Weeklies: | Balance: | |

Breakfast:

Snack:

Lunch:

Snack:

Supper:

Total:

Today:	Weeklies:	Balance:	

Breakfast:

Snack:

Lunch:

Snack:

Supper:

Total:

Today:	Weeklies:	Balance:	

Breakfast:

Snack:

Lunch:

Snack:

Supper:

Total:

Today: Weeklies: Balance:

Breakfast:

Snack:

Lunch:

Snack:

Supper:

Total:

Today:	Weeklies:	Balance:	

Breakfast:

Snack:

Lunch:

Snack:

Supper:

Total:

Today:	Weeklies:	Balance:	

Breakfast:

Snack:

Lunch:

Snack:

Supper:

Total:

Today:	Weeklies:	Balance:	

Breakfast:

Snack:

Lunch:

Snack:

Supper:

Total:

Today:	Weeklies:	Balance:	

Breakfast:

Snack:

Lunch:

Snack:

Supper:

Total:

Today:	Weeklies:	Balance:	

Breakfast:

Snack:

Lunch:

Snack:

Supper:

Total:

Today:	Weeklies:	Balance:

Breakfast:

Snack:

Lunch:

Snack:

Supper:

Total:

Today:	Weeklies:	Balance:

Breakfast:

Snack:

Lunch:

Snack:

Supper:

Total:

Today:	Weeklies:	Balance:

Breakfast:

Snack:

Lunch:

Snack:

Supper:

Total:

Today:	Weeklies:	Balance:	

Breakfast:

Snack:

Lunch:

Snack:

Supper:

Total:

Today:	Weeklies:	Balance:	

Breakfast:

Snack:

Lunch:

Snack:

Supper:

Total:

Today:	Weeklies:	Balance:	

Breakfast:

Snack:

Lunch:

Snack:

Supper:

Total:

| Today: | Weeklies: | Balance: |

Breakfast:

Snack:

Lunch:

Snack:

Supper:

Total:

<table>
<tr><td>Today:</td><td>Weeklies:</td><td>Balance:</td><td></td></tr>
</table>

Breakfast:

Snack:

Lunch:

Snack:

Supper:

Total:

| Today: | Weeklies: | Balance: |

Breakfast:

Snack:

Lunch:

Snack:

Supper:

Total:

Today:	Weeklies:	Balance:	

Breakfast:

Snack:

Lunch:

Snack:

Supper:

Total:

Today:	Weeklies:	Balance:

Breakfast:

Snack:

Lunch:

Snack:

Supper:

Total:

| Today: | Weeklies: | Balance: |

Breakfast:

Snack:

Lunch:

Snack:

Supper:

Total:

<table>
<tr><td>Today:</td><td>Weeklies:</td><td>Balance:</td></tr>
</table>

Breakfast:

Snack:

Lunch:

Snack:

Supper:

Total:

Today:	Weeklies:	Balance:	

Breakfast:

Snack:

Lunch:

Snack:

Supper:

Total:

Today:	Weeklies:	Balance:

Breakfast:

Snack:

Lunch:

Snack:

Supper:

Total:

Today:	Weeklies:	Balance:	

Breakfast:

Snack:

Lunch:

Snack:

Supper:

Total:

Today:	Weeklies:	Balance:

Breakfast:

Snack:

Lunch:

Snack:

Supper:

Total:

| Today: | Weeklies: | Balance: |

Breakfast:

Snack:

Lunch:

Snack:

Supper:

Total:

<table>
<tr><td>Today:</td><td>Weeklies:</td><td>Balance:</td></tr>
</table>

Breakfast:

Snack:

Lunch:

Snack:

Supper:

Total:

Today:	Weeklies:	Balance:	

Breakfast:

Snack:

Lunch:

Snack:

Supper:

	Total:	

Today:	Weeklies:	Balance:	

Breakfast:

Snack:

Lunch:

Snack:

Supper:

Total:

Today: Weeklies: Balance:

Breakfast:

Snack:

Lunch:

Snack:

Supper:

Total:

<table>
<tr><td>Today:</td><td>Weeklies:</td><td>Balance:</td><td></td></tr>
</table>

Breakfast:

Snack:

Lunch:

Snack:

Supper:

Total:

Today:	Weeklies:	Balance:	

Breakfast:

Snack:

Lunch:

Snack:

Supper:

Total:

Today:	Weeklies:	Balance:

Breakfast:

Snack:

Lunch:

Snack:

Supper:

Total:

Today:	Weeklies:	Balance:	

Breakfast:

Snack:

Lunch:

Snack:

Supper:

Total:

Today: Weeklies: Balance:

Breakfast:

Snack:

Lunch:

Snack:

Supper:

Total:

Today:	Weeklies:	Balance:	

Breakfast:

Snack:

Lunch:

Snack:

Supper:

Total:

Today: Weeklies: Balance:

Breakfast:

Snack:

Lunch:

Snack:

Supper:

Total:

Today:	Weeklies:	Balance:	

Breakfast:

Snack:

Lunch:

Snack:

Supper:

Total:

Today:	Weeklies:	Balance:	

Breakfast:

Snack:

Lunch:

Snack:

Supper:

Total:

Today:	Weeklies:	Balance:	

Breakfast:

Snack:

Lunch:

Snack:

Supper:

Total:

| Today: | Weeklies: | Balance: |

Breakfast:

Snack:

Lunch:

Snack:

Supper:

Total:

Today:	Weeklies:	Balance:	

Breakfast:

Snack:

Lunch:

Snack:

Supper:

Total:

Today: Weeklies: Balance:

Breakfast:

Snack:

Lunch:

Snack:

Supper:

Total:

| Today: | Weeklies: | Balance: | |

Breakfast:

Snack:

Lunch:

Snack:

Supper:

Total:

Today:	Weeklies:	Balance:

Breakfast:

Snack:

Lunch:

Snack:

Supper:

Total:

Today:	Weeklies:	Balance:	

Breakfast:

Snack:

Lunch:

Snack:

Supper:

Total:

Today:	Weeklies:	Balance:	

Breakfast:

Snack:

Lunch:

Snack:

Supper:

Total:

Today:	Weeklies:	Balance:	
Breakfast:			
Snack:			
Lunch:			
Snack:			
Supper:			
		Total:	

| Today: | Weeklies: | Balance: |

Breakfast:

Snack:

Lunch:

Snack:

Supper:

Total:

Today:	Weeklies:	Balance:	

Breakfast:

Snack:

Lunch:

Snack:

Supper:

Total:

| Today: | Weeklies: | Balance: |

Breakfast:

Snack:

Lunch:

Snack:

Supper:

Total:

| Today: | Weeklies: | Balance: | |

Breakfast:

Snack:

Lunch:

Snack:

Supper:

Total:

| Today: | Weeklies: | Balance: |

Breakfast:

Snack:

Lunch:

Snack:

Supper:

Total:

Today:	Weeklies:	Balance:	

Breakfast:

Snack:

Lunch:

Snack:

Supper:

Total:

Today:	Weeklies:	Balance:	

Breakfast:

Snack:

Lunch:

Snack:

Supper:

Total:

| Today: | Weeklies: | Balance: | |

Breakfast:

Snack:

Lunch:

Snack:

Supper:

Total:

Today:	Weeklies:	Balance:	

Breakfast:

Snack:

Lunch:

Snack:

Supper:

Total:

Today:	Weeklies:	Balance:	

Breakfast:

Snack:

Lunch:

Snack:

Supper:

Total:

Today:	Weeklies:	Balance:	

Breakfast:

Snack:

Lunch:

Snack:

Supper:

Total:

Today:	Weeklies:	Balance:	

Breakfast:

Snack:

Lunch:

Snack:

Supper:

Total:

| Today: | Weeklies: | Balance: |

Breakfast:

Snack:

Lunch:

Snack:

Supper:

Total:

Today:	Weeklies:	Balance:

Breakfast:

Snack:

Lunch:

Snack:

Supper:

Total:

| Today: | Weeklies: | Balance: | |

Breakfast:

Snack:

Lunch:

Snack:

Supper:

Total:

Today:	Weeklies:	Balance:	

Breakfast:

Snack:

Lunch:

Snack:

Supper:

Total:

| Today: | Weeklies: | Balance: | |

Breakfast:

Snack:

Lunch:

Snack:

Supper:

Total:

Today:	Weeklies:	Balance:	

Breakfast:

Snack:

Lunch:

Snack:

Supper:

Total:

Today:	Weeklies:	Balance:

Breakfast:

Snack:

Lunch:

Snack:

Supper:

Total:

9 781981 735921